Practical Record/Cumulative Record

for General Nursing and Midwifery Course

Practical Record/Cumulative Record
for General Nursing and Midwifery Course

Fourth Edition

I Clement
Doctorate of Philosophy in Nursing (PhD)
MSc Nursing (Medical Surgical Nursing) MA (Sociology) MSc (Psychology)
MBA (Education) MA (Child Care and Education) MA (Education) MPhil (Education)
Postgraduate (Hospital Administration)

Presently
Professor and Head
Department of Research and Development
RV College of Nursing
Bengaluru, Karnataka, India

Formerly
Principal and Professor
Department of Medical Surgical Nursing
Columbia College of Nursing
Bengaluru, Karnataka, India

Formerly, Principal
VSS College of Nursing
Bengaluru, Karnataka, India

PhD Guide, Examiner, Thesis Evaluator
Rajiv Gandhi University of Health Sciences
Bengaluru, Karnataka, India

Chief Editor for Nursing Journals
Editorial Chief for Various International Nursing Journals

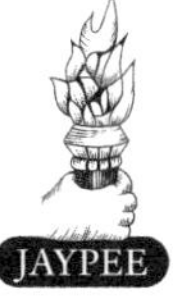

JAYPEE BROTHERS MEDICAL PUBLISHERS
The Health Sciences Publisher
New Delhi | London

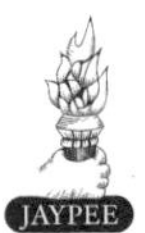

Jaypee Brothers Medical Publishers (P) Ltd

Headquarters
EMCA House
23/23-B, Ansari Road, Daryaganj
New Delhi 110 002, India
Landline: +91-11-23272143, +91-11-23272703
+91-11-23282021, +91-11-23245672
E-mail: jaypee@jaypeebrothers.com

Corporate Office
Jaypee Brothers Medical Publishers (P) Ltd.
4838/24, Ansari Road, Daryaganj
New Delhi 110 002, India
Phone: +91-11-43574357
Fax: +91-11-43574314
E-mail: jaypee@jaypeebrothers.com

Overseas Office
JP Medical Ltd.
83, Victoria Street, London
SW1H 0HW (UK)
Phone: +44-20 3170 8910
E-mail: info@jpmedpub.com

EU GPSR Authorised Representative
Logos Europe, 9 rue Nicolas Poussin
17000, La Rochelle, France
Phone: +33 (0) 6 67 93 73 78
E-mail: Contact@logoseurope.eu

Website: www.jaypeebrothers.com
Website: www.jaypeedigital.com

Inquiries for bulk sales may be solicited at: jaypee@jaypeebrothers.com

Practical Record/Cumulative Record for General Nursing and Midwifery Course

First Edition: 2008
Revised Reprint: 2009
Second Edition: 2016
Third Edition: 2019
Fourth Edition: 2022, **Reprint: 2025**
ISBN: 978-93-5465-239-4
Printed at: Samrat Offset Pvt. Ltd.

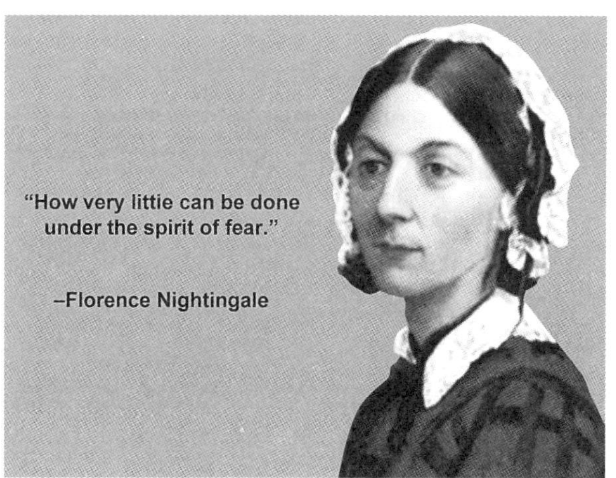

FLORENCE NIGHTINGALE

PIONEER OF MODERN NURSING

Born on: 12th May 1820 *Died on: 13th August 1910*

Nurses' Prayer

"AS I CARE
FOR MY PATIENTS TODAY
BE THERE WITH ME,
OH LORD, I PRAY.
MAKE MY WORDS KIND
AND IN MY HANDS
PLACE YOUR HEALING TOUCH.
LET YOUR LOVE SHINE
THROUGH ALL THAT I DO.
SO THOSE IN NEED
MAY HEAR AND FEEL YOU."

The Nightingale Pledge

I solemnly pledge myself before God and in the presence of this assembly, to pass my life in purity and to practice my profession faithfully. I will abstain from whatever is deleterious and mischievous, and will not take or knowingly administer any harmful drug. I will do all in my power to maintain and elevate the standard of my profession, and will hold in confidence all personal matters committed to my keeping, and all family affairs coming to my knowledge in the practice of my calling. With loyalty will I endeavor to aid the physician in his work, and devote myself to the welfare of those committed to my care.

PREFACE

It gives me immense pleasure to complete this task on fourth edition of *Practical Record/Cumulative Record for General Nursing and Midwifery Course*. First of all I would like to thank my Lord Almighty, for his kind blessings to complete this task. Nursing is a noble profession. Everyday nurses are facing different challenge in their daily work environment. There is need for every nursing professional to be updated with both theory knowledge and practical skills. Therefore, learning and demonstrating and practicing basic nursing procedures lay a strong foundation to sustain in the nursing profession to maintain its standard. Therefore, this practical record book serves as a legal tool as well as evidence for all nursing students not only to demonstrate but also practice the procedures until the students are confident enough to practice independently. This record book is prepared as per Indian Nursing Council (INC) syllabus, covers all the nursing procedures and it provides platform to learn and document the procedures done under supervision. I hope and wish all the nursing students best of luck whoever possess this book and follows the principles are sure to become competent nurse in future.

I Clement

GUIDELINES TO USE THE PRACTICAL RECORD

General Objectives

Nursing students will be able to understand, comprehend, develop skills in performing various procedures, following strictly related scientific principles and rationale for every step of nursing care, during their clinical postings in general and in speciality areas.

Contributory Objectives

In clinical postings, students will be able to:

1. Correlate the theory with practice in performing nursing procedures.
2. Demonstrate skills in performing the procedures accurately.
3. Assemble all the articles, required for procedure.
4. Develop skills in assessment, planning, implementing and evaluating the nursing care in all setup, i.e., hospital, community.
5. Perform all the nursing procedures based on scientific principles.
6. Perform procedures in systematic manner.

Instructions for Proper Use of Practical Record/Cumulative Record

1. Cumulative record serve as clinical evidence; therefore, it is the responsibility of the student to get signatures in the respective areas after completing the procedure with supervision of clinical instructors/nursing tutor.
2. Procedure demonstrated in the laboratories, to be signed by the staffs in demonstration column given, after completing the theory in the class, signatures to be given, only after doing redemonstration by students, conducting and viva with respective teachers.
3. Signatures to be given in the clinical demonstration columns in the clinicals, after performing at least 3 times each procedure followed by viva.
4. Signatures to be given in the respective columns with appropriate date.
5. A student who complete all the procedures signed both in demonstration and clinicals should submit to principal 2 weeks before university exams are only eligible for viva and practical examination each year and should ensure getting signatures from both internal and external examiners.
6. No student is allowed to duplicate signatures of staffs, if found, particular student will undergo a strict disciplinary action.
7. No student is permitted to do any procedure independently, but to do procedure under supervision for both clinical instructors/nursing tutor and ensure that he/she does to get signature.
8. Student is expected to take responsibility for her/his own learning by:
   a. Requesting the clinical instructor/nursing tutor to supervise a procedure she/he needs to have signature.
   b. Volunteering to do the procedure for experience she/he needs.
   c. Taking responsibility for obtaining signature from clinical instructor who has supervised procedure, immediately following the successful completion of a procedure.
9. Each staff can give only 25 signatures for each student, it should not exceed 25 signatures.
10. It is desirable that all procedures should be demonstrated in the laboratories/classrooms before they are carried out in the ward.
11. A student who lost the cumulative record, can replace the new one, he/she is responsible to get all the signatures back, teachers/institution will not take responsibility.
12. Signatures to be given in demonstration or in clinicals provided they do procedures and attend viva satisfactorily.
13. Cumulative record to be handled safely, covered neat, all the needed informations to be filled, passport size photograph to be fixed in the first page with signature of the student.
14. Students are not allowed to write and overwrite anything in the procedure book.
    All students are expected to take cumulative record for demonstration of laboratories and clinicals.
15. Students who repeat practical examinations should ensure that they get signatures from both internal and external examiner in the area provided for repeat.

STUDENT PROFILE

Passport Size Photo

Name of the Institution : ____________________

Address of the Institution : ____________________

Name of the Student (In BLOCK letters) : ____________________

Registration No. : ____________________

Date of Birth : ____________________

Age (in Years) : ____________________

Educational Qualification : ____________________

Father's Name : ____________________

Date of Joining the Course : ____________________

Date of Completion : ____________________

Permanent Address : ____________________

Signature of the Student:

Date:

Signature of the Principal:

Date:

COLLEGE SEAL

CONTENTS

COURSE DESCRIPTION
(Distribution of Weeks and Hours of the Course)

Total hours per week per student shall be 42 including classroom instruction and clinical practice

Year	*Weeks*		*Weeks (hours)*	*Total hours*
First year	Total weeks	52	46 weeks × 42 hours	1932
	Vacation	4		
	Examination preparation	1		
	Examinations	1		
	Functioning weeks	46		
Second year	Total weeks	52	46 weeks × 42 hours	1932
	Vacation	4		
	Examination preparation	1		
	Examinations	1		
	Functioning weeks	46		
Third year	Total weeks	52	First 6 months 24 weeks × 42 hours	1008
	Vacation	2		
	Examination preparation	1		
	Examinations	1	Second 6 months 24 weeks × 42 hours	1152
	Functioning weeks	48		
			Total hours	6024

FIRST YEAR

Theory: 655 **Practical: 1260**

Sl. No.	*Subjects*	*Theory*	*Practical*
1.	**Bioscience**	129	
	Anatomy and Physiology	90	
	Microbiology	30	
2.	**Behavioral Sciences**	65	
	Psychology	45	
	Sociology	20	
3.	**Nursing Foundation**	220	200 Laboratory and 724 Clinical
	Fundaments of Nursing	200	
	First Aid	20	
4.	**Community Health Nursing–I**	185	336
	Community Health Nursing	80	
	Environmental Hygiene	30	
	Health Education and Communication Skills	45	
	Nutrition	30	
5.	**English**	30	
6.	**Computer Education**	15	20
7.	**Co-curricular Activities**	20	
	Total hours	**655 hours**	**1280**
	Grand total		**1952**

SECOND YEAR

Theory: 420 **Practical: 1512**

Sl. No.	Subjects	Theory	Practical
1.	Medical Surgical Nursing–I	130	840
2.	Medical Surgical Nursing–II	130	
3.	Mental Health Nursing	70	336
4.	Child Health Nursing	70	336
5.	Co-curricular Activities	20	
	Total	420	1512
	Grand total		**1912**

THIRD YEAR: PART–I

Theory: 252 **Practical: 756**

Sl. No.	Subjects	Theory	Practical
1.	Midwifery and Gynecological Nursing	140	588
2.	Community Health Nursing–II	100	168
3.	Co-curricular Activities	12	
	Total	252	756
	Grand total		**1008**

THIRD YEAR: PART–II (INTEGRATED SUPERVISED INTERNSHIP)

Theory Hours

Sl. No.	Subjects	Hours
1.	Nursing Education	20
2.	Introduction to Research and Statistics	30
3.	Professional Trends and Adjustments	30
4.	Nursing Administration and Ward Management	40
	Total	**120**

Clinical Hours

Sl. No.	Subjects	Hours
1.	Medical Surgical Nursing	258
2.	Community Health Nursing	258
3.	Child Health Nursing	86
4.	Midwifery and Gynecological Nursing	344
5.	Mental Health Nursing	86
	Total	**1032**

SCHEME OF EXAMINATION

Sl. No.	Subjects	Total marks	Internal marks	External marks	Duration of exam
1.	**Bioscience**	100	25	75	3
	Anatomy and Physiology				
	Microbiology				
2.	**Behavioral Sciences**	100	25	25	3
	Psychology				
	Sociology				
3.	**Nursing Foundation**	100	25	25	3
	Fundaments of Nursing				
	First Aid				
4.	**Community Health Nursing–I**	100	25	25	3
	Community Health Nursing				
	Environmental Hygiene				
	Health Education and Communication Skills				
	Nutrition				
	PRACTICAL EXAMINATION Nursing Foundation	**100**	**50**	**50**	–

SECOND YEAR

Sl. No.	Subjects	Total marks	Internal marks	External marks	Duration of exam
1.	Medical Surgical Nursing–I	100	25	25	3
2.	Medical Surgical Nursing–II	100	25	25	3
3.	Mental Health Nursing	100	25	25	3
4.	Child Health Nursing	100	25	25	3
	PRACTICAL EXAMINATION				
1.	Medical Surgical Nursing–I and II	100	50	50	
2.	Mental Health Nursing	100	50	50	
3.	Child Health Nursing	100	50	50	

THIRD YEAR: PART–I

Sl. No.	Subjects	Total marks	Internal marks	External marks	Duration of exam
1.	Midwifery and Gynecological Nursing	100	25	25	3
2.	Community Health Nursing–II	100	25	25	3
	PRACTICAL EXAMINATION				
1.	Practical–I: Midwifery	100	50	50	
2.	Practical–II: Community Health Nursing	100	50	50	

THIRD YEAR: PART–II

Sl. No.	Subjects	Total marks	Internal marks	External marks	Duration of exam
1.	Nursing Education and Introduction to Research and Statistics	100	25	25	3
2.	Professional Trends and Adjustments in Nursing and Administration and Ward Management	100	25	25	3

General Nursing and Midwifery: Course Description

FIRST YEAR

Theory: 672 hours **Clinical: 1260 hours**

Sl. No.	*Subjects*	*Theory*	*Practical*
1.	**Biosciences**	**120**	
	• Anatomy and Physiology	90	
	• Microbiology	30	
2.	**Behavioral Sciences**	**65**	
	• Psychology	45	
	• Sociology	20	
3.	**Nursing Foundations**	**220**	**200—laboratory** **724—clinics**
	• Fundamentals of Nursing	200	
	• First Aid	20	
4.	**Community Health Nursing**	**185**	**336 hours**
	• Community Health Nursing	80	
	• Environmental Hygiene	30	
	• Health Education and Communication Skills	45	
	• Nutrition	30	
5.	**English**	**30**	
6.	**Computer Education**	**15**	
7.	**Co-curricular Activities**	**20**	
	Total	**672 (16 weeks)**	**1260 (30 weeks)**
	Grand Total		**1932**

SECOND YEAR

Theory: 420 hours **Clinical: 1512 hours**

Sl. No.	*Subjects*	*Theory*	*Practical*
1.	Medical Surgical Nursing–I	130	840 (24 weeks)
2.	Medical Surgical Nursing–II	130	
3.	Mental Health Nursing	70	336 (8 weeks)
4.	Child Health Nursing	70	336 (8 weeks)
	Co-curricular Activities	20	
	Total	**420 (10 weeks)**	**1512 (36 weeks)**
	Grand Total		**1932**

THIRD YEAR: PART–I

Theory: 252 hours **Clinical: 756 hours**

Sl. No.	*Subjects*	*Theory*	*Practical*
1.	Midwifery and Gynecological Nursing	140	588 (14 weeks)
2.	Community Health Nursing–II	100	168 (4 weeks)
3.	Co-curricular Activities	12	
	Total	**252**	**756**
	Grand Total		**1008**

THIRD YEAR: PART–II (INTEGRATED SUPERVISED INTERNSHIP)

Theory subjects:

Sl. No.	*Subjects*	*Hours*
1.	Nursing Education	20
2.	Introduction to Research and Statistics	30
3.	Professional Trends and Adjustments	30
4.	Nursing Administration and Ward Management	40
	Total	**120**

Clinical Areas

Sl. No.	*Clinical*	*Hours*
1.	Medical Surgical Nursing	258 (6 weeks)
2.	Community Health Nursing	258 (6 weeks)
3.	Child Health Nursing	86 (2 weeks)
4.	Midwifery and Gynecological Nursing	344 (8 weeks)
5.	Mental Health Nursing	86 (2 weeks)
	Total	**1032 (24 weeks)**

Night duty should be given in clinical area(s) in rotation.
* 43 hours per week for clinical and 5 hours per week for theory.
The students posted in the clinical areas should be accompanied by teaching faculty of the school.
The same practice must be followed when student are posted for requisite clinical experience to affiliated hospital/agency/institution.
The nursing service personnel must actively participate in supervising, guiding and evaluating students in the hospital wards, health centers and in the community.
1:10 teacher student ratio to be maintained during the supervised clinical practice.

SUMMARY OF TOTAL CLINICAL EXPERIENCES

Sl. No.	*Clinical*	*First Year*	*Second Year*	*Third Year-I*	*Third Year-II Internship*	*Total*
1.	Nursing Foundations	924 (22)				924 (22)
2.	Community Health Nursing	336 (8)		168 (4)	258 (6)	768 (18)
3.	Medical Surgical Nursing		840 (20)		258 (6)	1198 (26)
4.	Mental Health Nursing		336 (8)		86 (2)	412 (10)
5.	Child Health Nursing		336 (8)		86 (2)	412 (10)
6.	Midwifery and Gynecological Nursing			588 (14)	344 (8)	932 (21)

Scheme of Examination

FIRST YEAR

Paper	Subjects	Total Marks	Internal Marks	External Marks	Duration Examination
1.	**Biosciences** • Anatomy and Physiology • Microbiology	100	25	75	3
2.	**Behavioral Sciences** • Psychology • Sociology	100	25	75	3
3.	**Nursing Foundations** Fundamentals of Nursing First Aid	100	25	75	3
4.	**Community Health Nursing** • CHN–I • Environmental Hygiene • Health Education and Communication Skills • Nutrition	100	25	75	3
	Practical-I: Fundamentals of Nursing	100	50	50	-

SECOND YEAR

Paper	Subjects	Total Marks	Internal Marks	External Marks	Duration Examination
1.	Medical Surgical Nursing–I	100	25	75	3
2.	Medical Surgical Nursing–II	100	25	75	3
3.	Mental Health Nursing	100	25	75	3
4.	Child Health Nursing	100	25	75	3
	Practical Examination				
1.	Practical-I: Medical Surgical Nursing–I	100	50	50	-
2.	Practical-II: Child Health Nursing	100	50	50	
3.	Practical-III: Mental Health Nursing	100	50	50	
Note: * (only school examination, no council/board exam) *Practical examination for psychiatric nursing is to be conducted at the place of clinical experience at the end of clinical instruction by school, itself and marks shall be sent to the council/board.					

THIRD YEAR: PART–I

Paper	Subjects	Total Marks	Internal Marks	External Marks	Duration Examination
1.	Midwifery and Gynecological Nursing	100	25	75	3
2.	Community Health Nursing	100	25	75	3
	Practical Examination				
1.	Practical-I: Midwifery	100	50	50	–
2.	Practical-II: Community Health Nursing	100	50	50	

THIRD YEAR: PART–II (SCHOOL EXAMINATION)

Paper	Subjects	Total Marks	Internal Marks	External Marks	Duration Examination
1.	Nursing Education and Introduction to Research and Statistics	100	25	75	3
2.	Professional Trends and Adjustment, Nursing Administration and Ward Management	100	25	75	3

Examination Guidelines

1. Shall have one regular examination followed by supplementary examination in a year.
2. The candidates if fail in more than two subjects in any nursing program they can be promoted to next year.
3. A candidate can take any number of attempts with a condition that maximum period allowed is 6 years. However all papers need to be cleared before appearing in the final examination.
4. No institution shall submit student average internal marks more than 75% i.e., if 40 students are admitted in a course than the average score of the 40 students shall not exceed 75%. Example of 5 students: A = 25, B = 20, C = 22, D = 21, E = 24, Average score = 89.6%.
   This will not be accepted by the SNRC.

Eligibility for Admission to Examination

A candidate shall be eligible for the admission to the state council/board examination if the principle of the school certificate that:

1. She/he has completed not less than eleven months of the course.
2. She/he have attended 75% of the formal instructions given on each subject and 75% of the clinical field experience in each area/subject separately during the academic year, however, the total clinical/field experience prescribed must be completed before the final council/board examinations and before the issue of diploma.
   The diploma shall not be awarded to the student till she/he has completed the clinical/field requirements.
3. The overall performance of the student and her/his conduct during the entire academic year shall be satisfactory.
4. The student has passed in the internal assessment in each subject and practical(s).
5. The record of practical experience is complete.
   [The principle shall send to the council/board the internal assessment for each subject, i.e., both theory and practical (s) before the start of the examination along with the examination form].

Grading of Examination

Examination shall be graded on aggregate marks of the entire three and half years of the training program, as follows:

- Distinction—80% and above
- First division—70–79%
- Second division—60–69%
- Pass—50–59%

Theory Examination

1. Nursing teacher with minimum five years of teaching experience (recent) in a particular subject may be appointed as paper setters and examiners for that particular subject only.
2. Question paper should have a combination of essay, short answer and objective type question (situation based questions).
3. All units of a subject and sub-subject should be given due weightage in accordance with the instructional hours prescribed.

Practical Examination

1. Practical examination is to be conducted in the respective clinical area.
2. Nursing teacher with minimum of five years of teaching/clinical teaching experience in a particular subject/clinical area may be appointed as practical examiner.

EVALUATION

Internal Assessment

1. There shall be 25% internal assessment for all theory papers and 50% internal assessment for the entire practical.
2. A regular and periodic assessment for each subject and clinical/field experience is to be carried out.
3. For the purpose of internal assessment there shall be written test in each subject taken by the respective teacher each month.
   The student shall be required to maintain the practical record book and report of observation visits and diary for assessment must also be used. Marks shall be allotted for each of the following:
   a. Case study
   b. Case presentation
   c. Nursing care plan
   d. Maintenance of record books (procedure book and midwifery record book)
   e. Daily diary
   f. Area wise clinical assessment is to be carried out. Minimum two assessments are required in each clinical area.
4. Regular record of theory and practical is to be maintained. Task-oriented assessment is to be undertaken. Assessment shall be minted by teacher for each student each month. This can be checked by the council/board. Principal to sign all the records of examination. It should be displayed on the notice board for the information of the students.
5. A Candidate must secure 50% marks in internal assessment separately in each theory and practical. To be successful a student must get 50% marks in the internal as well as Council or Board Examination of each year.
6. For a student who appears for any supplementary examination her/his fresh internal assessment in the failed subject(s)/practical(s) is to be sent to the council/board.
7. State Nursing Council/Board should prepare a model perform for performance evaluation for each of the clinical area and circulate to all; schools of nursing for maintaining uniformity.

Each student is required to maintain the record of following assignment in clinical areas in each year:

First Year

a. Nursing care plan—4 in medical/surgical wards.
b. Daily diary—1 each in urban and rural community field.
c. Health—talk—1 each in urban and rural community field.
   Family study including—1 each in urban and rural community field.
   Health assessment of an—1 each in urban and rural community field.
   Individual in the family.
   Community profile—1 each in urban and rural community field.

Second Year

a. Medical Ward
   Nursing care plan—2
   Case study—1
   Case presentation—1
   Drug study—1
b. Surgical Ward
   Nursing care plan—2
   Case study—1
   Case presentation—1
   Drug study—1

c. Psychiatry Ward
   Nursing care plan—1
   Case study—1
   Case presentation—1
   Drug study—1
   Process recording—2
   Mental status examination—4

Third Year

a. Pediatric Ward
   Nursing care plan—2
   Case study—1
   Case presentation—1
   Drug study—1
   Observation report (newborn)—2
b. Maternity and Gynecological Ward
   Nursing care plan—2+1
   Case study—1+1
   Case presentation—1+1
   Drug study—1+1
c. Daily Diary Urban and Rural Community Field
   Health talk—2 each
   Family health nursing care plan—2 each
   Group project—1 each

In addition to above, each student shall maintain a procedure book and midwifery case book signed by concerned/supervisor and principle which is to be presented to examiner each year.

The above assignments are to be evaluated by concerned teachers for the purpose of internal assessment and shall be presented to the external examiner in a compiled form and it should be duly signed by her and should be stamped as cancelled after practical examination.

FIRST YEAR

NURSING FOUNDATIONS

Demonstration: 200 hours
Clinical: 724 hours

Sl. No.	*Subjects*	*Demonstration*		*Clinical*	
		Date	*Signature*	*Date*	*Signature*
1.	**Hospital Admission**				
	• Admission procedure				
	• Unit preparation for new patient				
	• Orientation of the unit				
	• Prepare admission bed				
	• Emergency admission				
	• Routine admission				
	• Transfer in/out/ interdepartmental				
	• Documentation of admission records				
2.	**Hospital Discharge**				
	• Discharge counseling				
	• Perform discharge procedure				
	• Planned discharge				
	• LAMA / DAMA				
	• Absconded				
	• Referrals and transfer out				
	• MLC cases				
	• Prepare patient records				
	• Disinfect the units				
	• Disinfect the equipment				
	• Terminal cleaning of the unit				
	• Documentation in discharge				
3.	**Nursing Process**				
	• History taking				
	• Nursing assessment				
	• Physical examination				
	• Nursing diagnosis				
	• Nursing planning				
	• Selection intervention				
	• Nursing evaluation				
	• Writing nursing care plan				
	• Application of critical thinking				

Sl. No.	Subjects	Demonstration		Clinical	
		Date	Signature	Date	Signature
	• Documentation in nursing process				
4.	**Communication**				
	• Verbal techniques				
	• Nonverbal techniques				
	• Interpersonal communication				
	• Therapeutic communication				
	• Skills and techniques used in communication				
	• Health talk with application of communication skills				
	• Patient teaching sessions				
5.	**Recording and Reporting**				
	• Documentation				
	• Change of shift reports				
	• Transfer reports				
	• Incident reports				
	• Patient report presentation				
	• Maintenance of records and reports				
	• Electronic recording system				
6.	**Check and Recording of Vital Signs**				
	• Temperature				
	a. Oral				
	b. Auxiliary				
	c. Rectal				
	d. Tympanal				
	• Pulse				
	• Respiration				
	• Blood pressure				
	• Pain				
	• Oxygen saturation				
	• Maintaining TPR sheet				
	• Recording vital signs				
	• Identifying deviated vitals				
7.	**Health Assessment**				
	• Health history taking				
	• Anthropometric measurements				
	• Check height of patient				
	• Check the weight of the patient				
	• General assessment				
	• Head-to-toe				
	• Methods of physical examination				

Sl. No.	Subjects	Demonstration		Clinical	
		Date	Signature	Date	Signature
	• Inspection				
	• Palpation				
	• Percussion				
	• Auscultation				
	• Manipulation				
	• Olfaction				
	• Interpreting the findings of physical examination				
	• Identifying the deviations through physical examinations				
	• Documentation in health assessment				
8.	**Patients Unit Preparations**				
	• Unit cleaning				
	• Prepare different types beds				
	• Open bed				
	• Closed bed				
	• Occupied bed				
	• Operation bed				
	• Amputation bed				
	• Cardiac bed				
	• Fracture bed				
	• Burns bed				
	• Divided bed				
	• Fowler bed				
	• Pain assessment and provision of comfort				
9.	**Comfort Devices**				
	• Extra pillows				
	• Back rest				
	• Cardiac table				
	• Sand bag				
	• Bed cradle				
	• Trochanter rolls				
	• Cotton ring and hand rolls				
	• Air cushion				
	• Water and air mattress				
	• Foot end elevator				
	• Knee rest				
	• Foot rest				
	• Trapeze bar				
	• Splints and braces				

Sl. No.	Subjects	Demonstration		Clinical	
		Date	Signature	Date	Signature
10.	**Safety Devices/Care**				
	• Restraints				
	• Protective padding				
	• Side rails and splints				
	• Safety belts				
	• Personal protective equipment (PPE)				
	• Discarding sharps and needles				
	• Documentation				
11.	**Hygienic Needs**				
	• Oral hygiene				
	• Assessment of neglected mouth				
	• Morning and evening care				
	• Bed bath and perineal care				
	• Assisted bed bath				
	• Care of pressure points				
	• Back care				
	• Hair care				
	• Skin care				
	• Bed shampoo or hair wash				
	• Pediculosis treatment				
	• Care of hand and feet				
	• Health education on personal, menstrual hygiene and environmental hygiene				
	• Documentation of the procedure				
12.	**Nutritional Needs**				
	• Nutritional assessment				
	• Oral feeding				
	• Nasogastric tube insertion and removal				
	• Nasogastric tube feeding				
	• Jejunostomy feeding				
	• Gastrostomy feeding				
	• Parenteral feeding—TPN				
	• Nasogastric suction/aspiration				
	• Nasogastric irrigation				
	• Planning and serving required type of therapeutic diet for patients				
	• Feeding the helpless patients				
	• Maintain the intake and output chart				

Sl. No.	Subjects	Demonstration		Clinical	
		Date	Signature	Date	Signature
	• Identifying deviations in the nutritional status				
	• Documentation of procedure				
13.	**Urinary Elimination**				
	• Assessment of urinary elimination				
	• Provides and removal of urinals/ bedpan				
	• Condom drainage				
	• Perineal care				
	• Catheterization male and female				
	• Catheter care				
	• Care of urinary drainage tubes				
	• Bladder irrigation				
	• Maintaining out chart				
	• Teaching: patient and family				
	• Identifying urinary problems				
	• Documentation of procedure				
14.	**Bowel Elimination**				
	• Assessment of bowel				
	• Provides bedpan				
	• Insertion of flatus tube				
	• Administration of enema				
	• Insertion of suppository				
	• Bowel wash				
	• Colonic irrigation				
	• Identify deviations in the bowel elemination				
	• Health teaching: patient and family				
	• Documentation of bowel elimination procedure				
15.	**Mobility and Exercise**				
	• Assessment of mobility				
	• Application of body mechanics principles in patient care				
	• Maintenance of body mechanics				
	• Maintain the body alignment and posture of the client				
	• Assist the client in ADLs, ambulation				
	• Perform range of motion exercises				
	• Deep breathing and coughing exercise				

Sl. No.	Subjects	Demonstration		Clinical	
		Date	Signature	Date	Signature
	• Changing position of helpless patient				
	• Transfer from bed to wheel chair and from wheel chair to bed				
	• Transfer from bed to stretcher and stretcher to bed				
	• Transfer from wheel chair to toilet seat and back to wheel chair				
	• Use of walker				
	• Use of crutches/canes				
	• Use of wheel chair				
	• Use of prosthetic devices				
	• Use side rails and restraints				
	• Log rolling				
	• Teaching patient and family				
	• Documentation of procedure				
16.	**Positions**				
	• Recumbent				
	• Lateral (right/left)				
	• Fowlers				
	• Cardiac				
	• Sims				
	• Roses				
	• C-shape				
	• Knee chest				
	• Lithotomy				
	• Prone				
	• Trendelenburg				
	• Jackknife position				
	• Maintaining position chart				
	• Care of pressure points				
17.	**Oxygen Administration**				
	• Pulse oximetry				
	• Methods of oxygen administration:				
	a. Mask				
	b. Catheters				
	c. Prongs/cannula				
	d. Tent				
	e. Oxygen hood				
	f. Venturi mask				
	g. Tracheostomy mask				

Sl. No.	Subjects	Demonstration		Clinical	
		Date	Signature	Date	Signature
	• AMBU bag				
	• Handling oxygen cylinders				
	• Humidification of oxygen				
	• Regulating oxygen by using flow meter				
	• Observation of oxygen toxicity				
	• Suctioning techniques:				
	a. Oropharyngeal suctioning				
	b. Nasopharyngeal suctioning				
	c. Endotracheal suctioning				
	d. Tracheostomy suctioning				
	• Care of oxygen cylinder				
	• Observation of oxygen toxicity				
	• Dry inhalations				
	• Moist inhalation				
	• Use of nebulizer				
	• Use of steam tent				
	• Use of Nelson inhaler				
	• Documentation in oxygen administration				
18.	**Therapeutic Procedures**				
	• Chest physiotherapy				
	• Postural drainage				
	• Care of chest drainage				
	• CPR—basic				
	• Intravenous therapy				
	• Blood transfusions				
	• Blood and blood component therapy				
	• Assisting various invasive procedures				
	• Documentation of procedure				
19.	**Specimen Collection**				
	• Urine—routine, culture and 24 hours				
	• Stool/feces—routine and culture				
	• Blood—routine, culture				
	• Peripheral blood smear				
	• Sugar—strip/glucometer				
	• Vomitus				
	• Throat swab				

Sl. No.	Subjects	Demonstration		Clinical	
		Date	Signature	Date	Signature
	• Urine test—reaction, specific gravity, albumin and sugar				
	• Nasal swab collection				
	• Safety measures in specimen collection				
	• Transporting specimens to laboratory				
	• Documentation in specimen collection				
20.	**Hot Applications**				
	• Hot water bag				
	• Hot fomentation				
	• Sitz bath				
	• Hot water bottles				
	• Chemical heating bottles				
	• Infrared rays				
	• Ultraviolet rays				
	• Heating lamps				
	• Electric heating pads				
	• Warm soaks (local baths)				
	• Documentation of procedures				
21.	**Cold Applications**				
	• Cold compress				
	• Ice cap				
	• Tepid sponge				
	• Cold sponging				
	• Use of cold drinks				
	• Chemical cold packs				
	• Documentation of procedures				
22.	**Care of Patient with Special Disability**				
	• Disability assessment				
	• Visually impaired				
	• Hearing impaired				
	• Mentally challenged				
	• Altered sensorium				
	• Care of patient with:				
	a. Fever				
	b. Dyspnea				
	c. Constipation and diarrhea				
	d. Fluid and electrolyte imbalance				

Sl. No.	Subjects	Demonstration		Clinical	
		Date	Signature	Date	Signature
	• Unconscious patient				
	• Recreational activities				
	• Diversional therapies				
23.	**Infection Control**				
	• Infection control measures				
	• Hand washing techniques				
	a. Medical hand washing				
	b. Surgical hand washing				
	• Preparation of isolation unit				
	• Practice techniques of wearing and removing personal protective equipment				
	• Disposal of waste				
	• Protocol and policies in infection control				
	• Barrier nursing				
24.	**Universal Precautions**				
	• Surgical wears				
	a. Mask				
	b. Gown				
	c. Gloves				
	d. Cap				
	e. Aprons				
	f. Shoes				
	g. Face shield or goggles				
	• Handling sharps and needles				
	• Biomedical waste management				
25.	**Decontamination of Equipment and Unit**				
	• Sterilization				
	• Handling sterilized equipment				
	• Calculate strengths of lotions				
	• Prepare lotions				
	• Preparing and packing articles for CSSD				
	• Assist in CSSD				
	a. Medical CSSD				
	b. Surgical CSSD				
	• Boiling of instruments				
	• Flaming				

Sl. No.	Subjects	Demonstration		Clinical	
		Date	Signature	Date	Signature
	• Hot air oven				
	• Chemical disinfection				
	• Aftercare of used sterilized equipment				
	• Ultrasonic disinfections				
	• Fumigation of unit				
26.	**Care of Equipment and Supplies**				
	• Needles and syringes				
	• Rubber goods				
	• Care of linens				
	• Care of rubber				
	• Care of furniture				
	• Care of enamel goods				
	• Care of glassware				
	• Care of sharp instrument				
27.	**Pre and Postoperative Care**				
	• Skin preparation of surgery				
	• Preparation of postoperative unit				
	• Pre and postoperative teaching, counseling and orientation				
	• Pre and postoperative exercises informed consent				
	• Pre and postoperative care				
	• Intraoperative care				
	• Pain management				
	• Care of surgical wound and dressing				
	• Care of surgical wound with drainage				
	• Suture care and removal				
	• Recovery room (PACU) care				
	• Teaching patient and family				
	• Identification of postoperative complications				
	• Documentation in perioperative care				
28.	**Medication Administration**				
	• Administration of medications in different forms and routes				
	• Oral, sublingual and buccal				
	• Intradermal				
	• Subcutaneous				

Sl. No.	Subjects	Demonstration		Clinical	
		Date	Signature	Date	Signature
	• Intramuscular				
	• Assist with intravenous medications				
	• Drug measurements and dose calculation				
	• Preparations of lotions and solutions				
	• Administers topical applications				
	• Insertion of drug into body cavity				
	a. Suppository				
	b. Medicated packs				
	• Instillation of medications and sprays				
	a. Ear				
	b. Nose				
	c. Eyes				
	d. Throat				
	e. Bladder				
	f. Vagina				
	g. Rectum				
	• Inhalation—moist and dry				
	• Medication error				
	• Documentation in medication administration				
29.	**First Aid and Bandaging**				
	• First aid assessment				
	• Prioritizing the care				
	• Principles and golden rule in first aid				
	a. Preparation of first aid kit				
	b. CPR				
	c. Snake bite				
	d. Dog bite				
	e. Stings				
	f. Accident/bleeding				
	g. Shock				
	h. Burns				
	i. Epistaxis's				
	j. Foreign body				
	k. Fracture				

Sl. No.	Subjects	Demonstration		Clinical	
		Date	Signature	Date	Signature
	l. Poisoning				
	m. Other emergencies				
	• Triage care				
	• Basic CPR (BLS)				
	• Documentation in first aid				
	• Bandaging				
	a. Simple spiral				
	b. Reverse spiral				
	c. Figure of eight				
	d. Head/Calpine				
	e. Eyes, ear, jaw, finger, elbow and knee				
	f. Use of triangular bandages				
	g. Use of slings				
	h. Use of binders				
30.	**Care of Death and Dying**				
	• Care of dying patient				
	• Handing over the body and valuables				
	• Caring and packing of dead body				
	• Transfer to mortuary with proper identification				
	• Counseling and supporting of grieving relatives				
	• Terminal care of the unit				
	• Postmortem				
	• Autopsy/embalming				
	• Documentation in first aid				
31.	**Observational Visit**				
	• Hospital				
	• Infection control unit				
	• CSSD				
	• Incineration unit				
32.	**Meeting Spiritual Needs of a Client**				
	• Spiritual assessment/care				
	• Arranging spiritual meetings with the client				
	• Assist in spiritual prayers				
	• Assist in client to gather the material related to spirituality				

Sl. No.	Subjects	Demonstration		Clinical	
		Date	Signature	Date	Signature
	• Spiritual counseling to patient and family				
33.	**Maintenance of Daily Clinical Diary**				

Nursing Care Plan

Sl. No.	Care Plan	Date	Signature
1.			
2.			
3.			
4.			
5.			

Demonstration of Physical Examination

Sl. No.		Date	Signature

Case Presentation/Ward Teaching

Sl. No.		Date	Signature
1.			
2.			
3.			
4.			

Health Education

Date	Topic	AV aids	Place	Individual/group	Signature

Signature of Class Coordinator

Signature of the Principal

COMMUNITY HEALTH NURSING – I

Theory: 185 hours
Community: 336 hours

		Demonstration in community laboratory		*Community*	
Sl. No.	*Subjects*	*Date*	*Signature*	*Date*	*Signature*
1.	**Orientation Visit to Urban and Rural Area**				
2.	**Mapping/Survey of Field Area:**				
	a. Numbering of houses				
	b. Urban				
	c. Rural				
3.	**Participate in Survey Activities:**				
	• Domiciliary				
	• Nutritional				
	• Sanitary				
4.	**Epidemiological Survey:**				
	• Morbidity survey				
	• Mortality survey				
5.	**Report Presentation: Urban and Rural**				
6.	**Prepare Community Profile**				
	• Individual and family:				
	a. Urban				
	b. Rural				
7.	**Perform Community Assessment**				
8.	**Perform Family Health Assessment**				
9.	**Perform Individual Health Assessment**				
10.	**Organize Home Visit**				
11.	**Preparation of Community Bag**				
12.	**Demonstrate Bag Technique**				
13.	**Develop and Maintain Rapport with Family**				
14.	**Identify the Health Needs and Problems In Community**				
15.	**Demonstrate Nursing Procedures**				
16.	**Make Referrals**				
17.	**Plan and Conduct Health Education on Identified Needs**				
18.	**Set up Clinic with Help of Staff**				
19.	**Maintain Records and Reports**				
20.	**Collect and Record Vital Health Statistics**				
21.	**Learn Various Organization of Community Health Importance**				
22.	**Assessment of Community Health Aspects of Nutrition In Family:**				

Sl. No.	Subjects	Demonstration in community laboratory		Community	
		Date	Signature	Date	Signature
	• Check height				
	• Check weight				
	• Check mid arm circumference				
	• Check chest circumference				
23.	**Identify the Health Needs of Various Age Groups**				
24.	**Assess the Community and the Family Environment**				
25.	**Maintain and Record Family Folders**				
26.	**Educate Community:**				
	• Nutrition disorder				
	• Food adulteration				
	• Breastfeeding				
	• Weaning				
27.	**Demonstrate Preparation and Methods of Cooking as per Nutritional Need of Family**				
28.	**Health Assessment Activities:**				
	• Urban				
	• Rural				
29.	**Health Education:**				
	• Individual				
	• Family				
	• Group				
	• Mass				
30.	**Prepare Appropriate AV Aids for Health Education**				
31.	**Meet the Specific Health Needs of Family:**				
	• Physical and hygienic needs				
	• Nutritional needs				
	• Elimination needs				
	• Psychological needs				
	• Spiritual needs				
32.	**Practice the Standards of Standing Orders of Community Nursing Practice**				
33.	**Treat the Minor Aliments**				
34.	**Implement Prescribed Treatments in Home**				
35.	**Administration of Medications in PHC/Subcenter/ CHC**				
	• Oral				
	• Intramuscular				
	• Assist intravenous infusion				
	• Subcutaneous				

Sl. No.	*Subjects*	*Demonstration in community laboratory*		*Community*	
		Date	*Signature*	*Date*	*Signature*
	• Intradermal				
	• Instillation of mediations in eye				
	• Instillation of mediations in ear				
	• Instillation of mediations in nose				
	• Eye irrigation				
	• Ear irrigation				
36.	**Urine Test**				
37.	**Assist in Implementation of:**				
	• National nutritional program				
	• National nutritional supplementation program				
	• Nutritional rehabilitation activities				
38.	**Vitamin A Supplements of Nutrition for Child under 3 Years**				
39.	**Assist for General Measures to Control and Prevent Communicable Disease**				

Sl. No.	*Observational visits*	*Date*	*Signature of supervisor*
1.	**Primary Health Center**		
2.	**Community Health Center**		
3.	**Subcenter**		
4.	**Anganwadi**		
5.	**Balawadi**		
6.	**Panchayat**		
7.	**Central Leprosarium**		
8.	**Water Purification Plant**		
9.	**Sewage Treatment Plant**		
10.	**Milk Diary**		

PRACTICAL EXAMINATION

Signature of Internal Examiner:

Date:

Signature of External Examiner:

Date:

Supplementary:

Signature of Internal Examiner:

Date:

Signature of External Examiner:

Date:

Supplementary:

Signature of Internal Examiner:

Date:

Signature of External Examiner:

Date:

NUTRITION PRACTICALS

Sl. No.	*Procedure*	*Date*	*Signature of supervisor*
1.	**Selection of Nutrients and Planning of Menu**		
2.	**Preservation and Storage of Foods**		
3.	**Preparation of Balanced Diet**		
4.	**Preparation of Weaning Diet**		
5.	**Therapeutic Diet:**		
	• High protein diet		
	• High calorie diet		
	• Salt restricted diet		
	• Low fat diet		
	• Low carbohydrate diet		
	• Fiber diet		
6.	**Preparation of Recipes:**		
	• Fluid diet:		
	• Tea/coffee		
	• Barley water		
	• Albumen water		
	• Lemon juice		
	• Egg flip		
	• Lassie		
	• Dhal soup		
	• Vegetable soup		
	• Meat soup		
	• Bone soup		
	• Butter milk		
	• Sago conjee		
	• Arrowroot conjee		
	• Orange juice		
	• Tomato soup		
	• Grape juice		
7.	**Light Diet:**		
	• Toast		
	• Porridge		
	• Salads		
	• Jelly		
	• Arrowroot		
	• Boiled egg		
	• Custard egg		
	• Scrambled egg		
	• Steamed fish		
	• Omelets		

Sl. No.	Procedure	Date	Signature of supervisor
	• Custards		
	• Rice kanji		
8.	**Vegetable Preparation:**		
	• Green leaf stuffed parota		
	• Vegetable biryani/rice		
	• Vegetable pachidies		
	• Vegetable cutlet		
9.	**Carbohydrates:**		
	• Rice kheer		
	• Idlies		
	• Rawa porridge		
	• Ragi porridge		
	• Rawa upma		
	• Wheat payasam		
	• Banana milk shake		
10.	**Proteins:**		
	• Sprouted grams salads		
	• Groundnut milkshakes		
	• Fish curry		
	• Fish fry		
	• Meat curry		
	• Vada		
	• Dhal curry		
	• Channa dhal curry		
	• Soybean cutlet		
	• Vermicelli payasam		
11.	**Fats:**		
	• Paneer mutter masala		
	• Poories		
	• Bread cheese sandwich		
	• Potato bonda		
12.	**Practice Different Methods of Cooking:**		
	• Boiling		
	• Baking		
	• Steaming		
	• Frying		
	• Simmering		
	• Grilling		
	• Roasting		
	• Stewing		
13.	**Completed the Demonstration of Nutrition Practical**		

OBSERVATION VISIT

Sl. No.	*Place of visit*	*Date*	*Signature of supervisor*
1.	CFTRI		
2.	Food Preservation and Storage Centers		
3.	Food Processing Agency		
4.	Local Food Preparation Units		
5.	Food Fortification Centers		
6.	Nutritional Rehabilitation Center		
7.	Milk Diary		
8.	Dietary Units in Hospital		
9.	Food Sanitation Units		
10.	Slaughter House		

SECOND YEAR

MEDICAL SURGICAL NURSING

Theory: 260 hours
Clinical: 840 hours

Sl. No.	*Subjects*	*Demonstration*		*Clinical*	
		Date	*Signature*	*Date*	*Signature*
1.	**Assessment of Patient:**				
	• History taking				
	• Physical examination				
	• Methods:				
	a. Inspection				
	b. Palpation				
	c. Auscultation				
	d. Percussion				
	e. Manipulation				
	f. Olfaction				
	• Perform general and specific examination				
	• Identify the alteration and deviations				
	• Documentation in physical examination				
	• Practice medical surgical safety measures				
	• Practice standard safety measures				
2.	**Medication Administration:**				
	• Oral				
	• Sublingual				
	• Intradermal				
	• Subcutaneous				
	• Topical/spray				
	• Intravenous cannulation				
	• Intravenous infusion				
	• Intravenous calculation				
	• Parenteral therapy—TPN				
	• Maintain intake output chart				
	• Intramuscular				
	• Administration of drugs by:				
	a. Infusion pump				
	b. Epidural				
	c. Intrathecal				
	d. Intracardiac				

Sl. No.	Subjects	Demonstration		Clinical	
		Date	Signature	Date	Signature
3.	**Therapeutic Procedures:**				
	• Oxygen therapy in different methods				
	• Endotracheal suctioning				
	• Ventilator				
	• Nebulization				
	• Chest physiotherapy				
	• Nasogastric (NG) tube feeding				
	• Blood component therapy				
	• Catheterization—male				
	• Catheterization—female				
	• Bladder irrigation				
	• Bowel wash				
	• Enema				
	• Colostomy irrigation				
	• Catheter care				
	• Dialysis:				
	a. Hemodialysis				
	b. Peritoneal				
4.	**Diagnostic Procedures**:				
	• Electrocardiogram				
	• Doppler studies				
	• Central venous pressure				
	• Abdominal paracentesis				
	• Lumbar puncture				
	• Gastric lavage				
	• Sternal puncture				
	• Thoracocentesis				
	• Cystoscopy				
	• Cystometrogram				
	• Intravenous pyelogram and KUB				
	• Barium enema				
	• Renal biopsy				
	• Liver biopsy				
	• Proctoscopy				
	• Endoscopy				
	• Cholecystography				
	• Esophagogastroduodenoscopy				
	• Blood studies				
	• Thyroid studies				
	• FBS/PBBS/RBS				

Sl. No.	Subjects	Demonstration		Clinical	
		Date	Signature	Date	Signature
	• Glucose tolerance test				
	• Liver function test				
	• Pulmonary function test				
5.	**Pre and Postoperative Nursing Care**				
	• Preoperative nursing				
	• Skin preparation:				
	a. Local surgery				
	b. General surgery				
	• Physical preparation				
	• Psychological preparation				
	• Informed consent				
	• Spiritual preparation				
	• Intraoperative nursing				
	• PACU/Recovery room care				
	• Setting up postoperative unit				
	• Postoperative care:				
	a. Immediate postoperative care				
	b. Late postoperative care				
	• Identifying postoperative complications				
	• Care of wound and drainage				
	• Suture removal				
	• Early ambulation and postoperative exercise				
	• Care of chest drainage				
	• Ostomy care:				
	a. Colostomy care				
	b. Gastrostomy care				
	• Blood and its component therapy				
	• Practice universal precautions				
6.	**Operation Theater Nursing:**				
	• Packing of articles for surgery				
	• Surgical hand washing				
	• Surgical scrubbing				
	• Glowing				
	• Gowning				
	• Use of mask, cap and goggles				
	• Identify instruments used for common surgeries				
	• Maintain operation instrument book				
	• Identify suture material used for common surgery				

Sl. No.	Subjects	Demonstration		Clinical	
		Date	Signature	Date	Signature
	• Disinfection of OT				
	• Carbolization				
	• Fumigation				
	• Preparation of instruments sets of common operations				
	• Setting up of trolley for surgery				
	• Sterilization of sharp and other instruments				
	• Preparation of OT table				
	• Positioning for surgery				
	• Assisting in anesthesia				
	• Circulatory nurse—monitoring the patient				
	• Endotracheal intubation				
	• Handling specimen				
	• Disposal of waste as per the guidelines				
	• Assisting in major surgeries:				
	1.				
	2.				
	3.				
	4.				
	5.				
	• Assisting in minor surgeries:				
	1.				
	2.				
	3.				
	4.				
	5.				
	• Equipment used in OT				
	• Monitoring the patient in OT				
	• OT equipment count before and after surgery—checklist				
7.	**Nursing Care of Patient in ICU**				
	• Monitoring patient in ICU				
	• Maintain ICU flowchart				
	• Care of patient in ventilator				
	• Perform endotracheal intubation				
	• Demonstrate the uses of:				
	a. Ventilator				
	b. Cardiac monitors				
	c. Infusion pumps				
	d. ABG machines				
	e. Interpret ABG analysis				

Sl. No.	Subjects	Demonstration		Clinical	
		Date	Signature	Date	Signature
	f. Pulse oximeter				
	g. Defibrillator/AEB				
	• Assist with ICU procedures:				
	a. CVP line				
	b. Arterial line				
	c. Endotracheal intubation/extubation				
	d. Endotracheal suctioning				
	e. Tracheostomy				
	f. Chest tube				
	g. Pace maker				
	h. AMBU bag ventilation				
	• Perform CPR				
	• Crash cart				
	• Preparation of emergency trolley crash cart				
	• Administration of ICU drugs:				
	a. Infusion pumps				
	b. Epidural				
	c. Intravenous				
	d. Intrathecal				
	• Chest physiotherapy				
	• Perform active and passive exercise				
	• Counseling for patient and family with grief and bereavement				
8.	**Geriatric Nursing:**				
	• Assessment—head to toe				
	• Identify health problems:				
	a. Physical				
	b. Psychological/emotional				
	c. Social				
	d. Spiritual				
	• Care of sick elderly				
	• Geriatric counseling				
9.	**Nursing Care of Patient with Cancer:**				
	• Assessment of warning signs				
	• TNM classifications				
	• Self-breast examination				
	• Assist in diagnostic procedures:				
	a. Biopsy				
	b. Pap smear				

Sl. No.	Subjects	Demonstration		Clinical	
		Date	Signature	Date	Signature
	c. Bone marrow aspiration				
	d. Mammography				
	• Assist in therapeutic procedures				
	• Participate in various modalities of treatment:				
	a. Chemotherapy				
	b. Radiotherapy				
	c. Pain therapy				
	d. Stoma care				
	e. Brachy therapy				
	f. Hormonal therapy				
	g. Gene therapy				
	h. Alternative therapy				
	• Participate in palliative care				
	• Counsel and teach patient's families				
10.	**Nursing Care of Patient with Burns**				
	• Burns assessment: Rule of nine				
	• Calculation of percentage and degree of burns				
	• Calculation of fluid and electrolyte therapy:				
	a. Assess				
	b. Calculate				
	c. Replace				
	• Record intake output chart				
	• Care of burn wounds				
	• Bathing burns/hydrotherapy				
	• Burns dressing				
	• Perform active and passive exercises				
	• Practice medical and surgical asepsis				
	• Assist in reconstruction surgeries				
	• Teach patients and families				
	• Participate in rehabilitation program				
	• Nursing care of patient with dermatology				
	• Administer topical medications				
	• Give medicated baths				
11.	**Nursing Care of Patient with Eye Disorders**				
	• Examination of eye				

Sl. No.	Subjects	Demonstration		Clinical	
		Date	Signature	Date	Signature
	• Assist in diagnostic procedures:				
	a. Fundoscopy				
	b. Retinoscopy				
	c. Ophthalmoscopy				
	d. Refraction test				
	e. Visual acuity				
	f. Tonometry				
	g. Syringing				
	• Ophthalmic emergencies				
	a. Foreign body removal				
	b. Retinal detachment				
	c. Sore eye				
	• Perform/assist in irrigation				
	• Application of ointments				
	• Application of eye bandage				
	• Pre and postoperative care of eye surgeries				
	Teach patients and families				
12.	**Nursing Care of Patient with ENT Disorders**				
	• Examination of ear, nose and throat				
	• Assisting with diagnostic procedures:				
	a. Speech test				
	b. Tuning fork: Rinne and Weber test				
	c. Finger friction test				
	d. Audiometric test				
	e. Tympanometry				
	f. Throat swab culture				
	g. Caloric test				
	• Installation of drops				
	• Application of ointments				
	• Perform/assist irrigations				
	• Assist in removal of foreign bodies				
	• Application of ear bandage				
	• Tracheostomy care				
	• Pre and postoperative care of ENT surgeries				
	• Teach patients and families				
13.	**Nursing Care of Patients with Cardiac Disorders**				
	• Cardiac assessment				

Sl. No.	Subjects	Demonstration		Clinical	
		Date	Signature	Date	Signature
	• Physical examination				
	• Electrocardiogram				
	• Assisting diagnostic procedures				
	a. Electrocardiogram				
	b. Stress ECG				
	c. Echocardiogram invasive				
	d. Cardiac catheterization				
	e. Cardiac enzymes				
	f. Central venous pressure				
	g. Pulmonary artery wedge pressure				
	• Administrator cardiac drugs				
	• Assisting therapeutic procedures:				
	a. Percutaneous transluminal coronary angioplasty				
	b. Thrombolytic therapy				
	• Cardiac surgeries				
	a. Open heart surgeries				
	b. Closed heart surgeries				
	c. Heart transplantation				
	• Cardiac rehabilitation				
	• Cardiopulmonary resuscitation				
	• Teach patients and families				
	• Practice medical and surgical asepsis				
	• Standard safety measures				
14.	**Nursing Care of Patients with Skeletal-Muscular Disorders**				
	• Orthopedic assessment				
	• Physical examination				
	• Assist in application and removal of plaster cast				
	• Application of traction:				
	a. Skin traction				
	b. Bucks extension traction				
	c. Cervical Traction				
	d. Skeletal traction				
	• Assist in application and removal of prosthesis				
	• Physiotherapy:				
	a. Range of motion exercises				

Sl. No.	Subjects	Demonstration		Clinical	
		Date	Signature	Date	Signature
	b. Muscle strengthen exercises				
	c. Crutch maneuvering technique				
	• Assist with walking aids:				
	a. Canes				
	b. Walkers				
	c. Crèches				
	• Activities of daily living				
	• Ambulation				
	• Teach and counsel patients and families				
	• Stump care				
15.	**Nursing Care of Patient with Communicable Diseases**				
	• Assessment of patients with communicable diseases				
	• Use of personal protective equipment (PPE) and barrier nursing				
	• Health teaching for prevention of infectious diseases				
	• Counseling of HIV/AIDS patients				
	• Counseling of family members				
16.	**Nursing Care of Adult Patient in Emergency and Disaster Situation**				
	• Practice triage				
	• Code blue/green/red				
	• Assist causalities:				
	a. Assessment				
	b. Examination				
	c. Investigation				
	d. Implementation of care				
	• Assist in legal practices/procedures during emergencies				
	• Standing orders/protocols				
	• Maintenance of recording in emergency situation				
	• Counseling of family members during grief and bereavement				

Nursing Care Plan

Sl. No.	Care Plan	Date	Signature
1.			
2.			
3.			
4.			
5.			

Demonstration of Physical Examination

Sl. No.		Date	Signature

Case Presentation/Ward Teaching

Sl. No.		Date	Signature
1.			
2.			
3.			
4.			

Health Education

Date	Topic	AV aids	Place	Individual/group	Signature

Signature of Class Coordinator **Signature of the Principal**

MENTAL HEALTH NURSING

Theory: 70 hours
Clinical: 336 hours

		Demonstration		*Clinical*	
Sl. No.	***Subjects***	***Date***	***Signature***	***Date***	***Signature***
1.	**Assessment of Patients with Mental Health Problems**				
	• History taking				
	• Perform mental status examination				
	• Mini mental status examination				
	• Neurological examination				
	• Psychological testing				
	• Psychometric assessment				
	• Physical investigation:				
	a. CT scan				
	b. MRI				
	c. EMG				
	d. EEG				
2.	**Psychiatric Admission and Discharge**				
	• Voluntary admission				
	• Involuntary admission				
	• Emergency admission				
	• Temporary admission				
	• Admission and discharge of criminal lunatics				
	• Reception order				
	• Assist in therapeutic modalities				
	• Physical therapy				
3.	**Electroconvulsive Therapy**				
	• Care before ECT				
	• Care during ECT				
	• Care after ECT				
4.	**Psychotherapies**				
	• Behavior therapy				
	• Milieu therapy				
	• Aversion therapy				
	• Group therapy				
	• Hypnosis				
	• Psychoanalysis				
	• Family therapy				
	• Diversion therapy				
	• Individual psychotherapy				

Sl. No.	Subjects	Demonstration		Clinical	
		Date	Signature	Date	Signature
	• Music therapy				
	• Recreation therapy				
	• Play therapy				
	• Occupational therapy				
	• Dance therapy				
5.	**Psychopharmacological Therapy**				
	• Lithium therapy				
	• Narcoanalysis				
	• Disulfiram therapy				
6.	**Assessment of Children with Various Mental Health Problems**				
	• History taking				
	• Assist in psychometric assessment				
	• Observe and assist in various therapies				
7.	**Care of Child with Mental Retardation**				
8.	**Care of Child Psychiatric Disorders**				
9.	**Health Educate and Teach Family and Significant others**				
10.	**Maintain Therapeutic Communication**				
11.	**Process Recording**				
12.	**Prepare Patients for Activities of Daily Living**				
13.	**Administration of Psychiatric Medications**				
14.	**Nursing Care of Clients with:**				
	• Schizophrenia				
	• Organic brain disorders				
	• Mood disorders				
	• Psychiatric emergencies				
	• Neurotic disorders				
	• Substance abuse/deaddiction				
15.	**Participation in Community Mental Health services**				

Sl. No.	Clinical area	Diagnosis	Date of submission	Signature of clinical supervisor
1.	**History Collection Psychiatric OPD**			
2.	**History Collection in Female Open Psychiatric Ward**			
3.	**History Collection in Male Open Psychiatric Ward**			
4.	**Mental Status Examination in OPD**			

Sl. No.	Clinical area	Diagnosis	Date of submission	Signature of clinical supervisor
5.	History collection and Mental Status Examination in Closed Ward for Male Patient			
6.	History Collection and Mental Status Examination in Closed Ward for Female Patient			
7.	History Collection and Mental Status Examination in Child Guidance Clinic			
8.	Report on Observation of Activities in OPD			
9.	Process Recording—Male Patient			
10.	Process Recording—Female Patient			

Health Education to Family

Sl. No.	Topic	AV aids used	Date	Signature of supervisor

Care Study (Five Days Care) and Presentation of Case

Sl. No.	Clinical area	Diagnosis	Date of submission	Date of presentation	Signature of supervisor

Care Plan: Three Days Care (Psychosis-1, Neurosis-1 and Drugs/alcohol Addiction-1)

Sl. No.	Clinical area	Diagnosis	Date of care started	Date of submission	Signature of supervisor
1.					
2.					
3.					

Drug Book

Sl. No.	Date of submission	Signature of supervisor
1.		
2.		

Observational Report

Sl. No.	Place of visits	Date of visit	Date of submission of observation report	Signature of supervisor
1.	Child guidance clinic			
2.	Day care center			
3.	Rehabilitation center			
4.	Community psychiatric rehabilitation center			

Signature of Class Coordinator **Signature of the Principal**

CHILD HEALTH NURSING

Theory: 70 hours
Clinical: 336 hours

		Demonstration		*Clinical*	
Sl. No.	*Subjects*	*Date*	*Signature*	*Date*	*Signature*
1.	**Nursing Care of Children with Medical Disorders**				
2.	**Pediatric History/Physical Examination**				
3.	**Administration of Medication:**				
	• Oral				
	• Intramuscular				
	• Intravenous				
	• Subcutaneous				
	• Suppositories				
	• Intradermal injection				
	• Instillation of medications in eye				
	• Instillation of medications in nose				
	• Instillation of medications in ear				
	• Calculation of fluid replacements				
	• Prepare different strengths of IV fluids				
	• Topic application				
	• Documentation in medication administration				
4.	**Restraints:**				
	• Elbow restraints				
	• Mummy restraints				
	• Jacket restraints				
	• Clove hitch restraints				
	• Use of splints				
	• Mitten/finger restraints				
	• Abdominal restraints				
	• Crib-net restraint				
	• Safety belt				
5.	**Oxygen Therapy:**				
	• Tent				
	• Oxyhood				
	• Nasal catheter				
	• Nasal cannula				
	• Mask				
	• AMBU bag				
	• Ventilator				

Sl. No.	Subjects	Demonstration		Clinical	
		Date	Signature	Date	Signature
6.	**Feeding Children by:**				
	• Katori and spoon				
	• Formula preparation				
	• Breastfeeding				
	• Weaning				
	• NG tube feeding				
	• Cleaning and sterilization of feeding				
	• Complementary feeding				
	• Supplementary feeding				
7.	**Specimen Collection:**				
	• Urine: Culture and sensitivity				
	• Stool				
	• Blood studies				
	• Sputum for culture				
	• Throat swab				
	• Skin scraping				
	• Assist with common diagnostic procedures				
	• Assist with common therapeutic procedures				
8.	**Teach Mothers/Parents:**				
	• Malnutrition				
	• Oral rehydration therapy				
	• Feeding and weaning				
	• Immunization schedule				
	• Play therapy for different age groups				
	• Specific disease conditions				
9.	**Nursing Care of Children with Surgical Disorders**				
10.	**Calculate and Prepare and Administer IV Fluids**				
11.	**Bowel Wash**				
12.	**Care of Ostomies and Irrigation:**				
	• Colostomy				
	• Ureterostomy				
	• Gastrostomy				
13.	**Urinary Catheterization and Drainage**				
14.	**Feeding:**				
	• Nasogastric				

Sl. No.	*Subjects*	*Demonstration*		*Clinical*	
		Date	*Signature*	*Date*	*Signature*
	• Gastrostomy				
	• Jejunostomy				
	• Feeding child with cleft lip and cleft palate				
15.	**Surgical Care:**				
	• Preoperative care				
	• Postoperative care				
	• Surgical wounds				
	• Surgical dressing				
16.	**Perform Assessment of Children:**				
	• Health, developmental and anthropometric: Newborn				
	• Record APGAR				
17.	**Immediate Care of Newborn:**				
	• Cord care				
	• Eye care				
	• Baby bath				
	• Rooming-in				
	• Head to toe physical assessment				
	• Neurological assessment				
	• Reflexes				
18.	**Care of Child in NICU:**				
	• Care of child in PICU				
	• Incubator care				
	• Phototherapy				
	• Radiant warmer				
	• Care of preterm				
	• Care of low birth weight baby				
	• Care of high risk newborn				
	• Care of child in ventilator				
	• Exchange transfusion				
19.	**Infant—Assessment of Growth and Assessment:**				
	• Assist in preparation of weaning diet				
	• Nutrition counseling				
	• Immunization of infant				
	• Meet the play needs				
	• Prevention of accidents				

Sl. No.	Subjects	Demonstration		Clinical	
		Date	Signature	Date	Signature
20.	**Toddler—Assessment of Growth and Assessment:**				
	• Assist in preparation of menu plan and diet				
	• Nutrition counseling				
	• Immunization of toddler				
	• Meet the play needs				
	• Prevention of accidents				
	• Assist the child for toilet training				
21.	**Preschooler—Assessment of Growth and Assessment**				
	• Assist in preparation of menu plan and diet				
	• Nutrition counseling				
	• Immunization of preschooler				
	• Meet the play needs				
	• Assist the child and parent in prevention of accidents				
22.	**School Age—Assessment of Growth and Assessment:**				
	• Assist in preparation of menu plan and diet				
	• Nutrition counseling				
	• Immunization of child of school age				
	• Meet the play needs				
	• Assist the child and parent in prevention of accidents				
	• Carry out sex education activities				
23.	**Assessment of Sick Child:**				
	• Admission of sick child				
	• Preparation for diagnostic test				
	• Collection of specimen				
24.	**Care of Child with:**				
	• Congenital defects				
	• CNS diseases				
	• Cardiovascular disorders				
	• Respiratory disorders				
	• GI disorders				
	• Musculoskeletal disorders				
	• Renal disorders				
	• Behavioral disorders				
	• Physically challenged				
	• Menstrual problems				

Sl. No.	Subjects	Demonstration		Clinical	
		Date	Signature	Date	Signature
25.	**Participation in:**				
	• Immunization activities				
	• School health activities				
	• RCH Programme activities				
	• CSSM Programme activities				
	• National nutritional programmes				
	• Under five children approach				
	• Teach milestones of all age group to parents				

Observational Visits

Sl. No.	Place of visit	Date	Clinical supervisor signature
1.	**Child Guidance Clinic**		
2.	**MCH Clinic**		
3.	**Under Five Clinic**		
4.	**Well Baby Clinic**		
5.	**Anganwadi**		
6.	**Balawadi**		
7.	**Guidance and Counseling Center**		
8.	**ICDS Center**		
9.	**Baby Friendly Hospital**		
10.	**Child Welfare Agencies:**		
	• Juvenile delinquent homes		
	• Crèche		
	• Play home		
	• Handicapped homes		
	• Nursery school		
	• Nutritional child clinic		

Nursing Care Plan

Sl. No.	Clinical area	Care Plan	Date	Signature of supervisor
1.	Pediatric medical ward			
2.	Pediatric surgical ward			

Case Study and Case Presentation

Sl. No.	Clinical area	Date of submission	Date of case presentation	Signature of supervisor
1.	Pediatric medical ward			
2.	Pediatric surgical ward			

Health Education

Sl. No.	*Clinical area*	*Date of submission*	*Date of health education*	*Signature of supervisor*
1.	Pediatric medical ward			
2.	OPD/immunization/adolescent clinic			

Drug Book

Sl. No.	*Date of submission of drug book*	*Signature of supervisor*
1.	Pediatric medical ward	
2.	Pediatric surgical ward	
3.	PICU	
4.	NICU	
5.	OPD	

PRACTICAL EXAMINATION

MEDICAL SURGICAL NURSING

Signature of Internal Examiner

Date:

Signature of External Examiner

Date:

Supplementary

Signature of Internal Examiner

Date:

Signature of External Examiner

Date

MENTAL HEALTH NURSING

Signature of Internal Examiner

Date:

Signature of External Examiner

Date:

Supplementary

Signature of Internal Examiner

Date:

Signature of External Examiner

Date:

CHILD HEALTH NURSING

Signature of Internal Examiner

Date:

Signature of External Examiner

Date:

Supplementary

Signature of Internal Examiner

Date:

Signature of External Examiner

Date:

THIRD YEAR

MIDWIFERY AND GYNECOLOGICAL NURSING

Theory: 140 hours
Clinical: 588 hours

Sl. No.	*Subjects*	*Demonstration*		*Clinical*	
		Date	*Signature*	*Date*	*Signature*
1.	**Setting up of Prenatal Unit:**				
	• Assessment of pregnant women				
	• Antenatal history taking				
	• Preconception counseling				
	• Physical examination				
	• Abdominal examination				
	• Identify deviations in prenatal examination				
	• Calculating expected date of delivery (EDD/LMP)				
	• Diagnose pregnancy using pregnancy detection kit (preg-card)				
	• Invasive antenatal diagnostic test				
	• NST/OCT/USG/TVS				
	• Antenatal diet				
	• Antenatal exercises				
	• Antenatal immunization				
	• Maintenance of antenatal records				
2.	**Recording of:**				
	• Vital signs				
	• Weight				
	• Height				
	• Blood pressure				
	• Hemoglobin				
	• Urine: Sugar and albumin				
3.	**Antenatal Care**:				
	• Antenatal examination/identification of high risk ANC				
	• Inspection head to toe examination of the mother				
	• Examination of breast and nipple				
	• Examination of the abdomen:				
	a. Inspection				
	b. Measure the abdominal girth and fundal height				
	c. Estimate the gestational age				
	d. Palpation—fundal, lateral and pelvic examination				

Sl. No.	Subjects	Demonstration		Clinical	
		Date	Signature	Date	Signature
	• Assessment of risk status				
	• Setting up of eclamptic unit				
	• Immunization				
	• Teaching antenatal mothers				
	• Maintenance of antenatal records				
4.	**Assessment of Women in Labor:**				
	• Assist in setting labor room				
	• Setting up of newborn resuscitation unit				
	• Skin and perineal preparation				
	• Administration of enema before labour				
	• Assessment of women in labor				
	• Assist in induction of labor:				
	a. Medical				
	b. Surgical				
	• Per-vaginal examination				
	• Maintenance of partograph				
	• Monitoring and caring of women in labor				
	• Perineal preparation of mother for labor				
5.	**Monitoring and Recording Uterine Contraction and Relaxation Chart:**				
	• Monitoring and recording of FSH-cardiotocography				
	• Monitoring and recording of cervical dilatation and fetal descent				
	• Conducting normal deliveries				
	• Administration of uterotonic drugs—oxytocin and misoprostol				
	• Epidural analgesia				
	• Administration of anticonvulsants and antihypertensive drugs				
	• Examination of placenta				
	• Episiotomy and suturing				
	• Maintenance of labor and birth records				
6.	**Assist in Deliveries with Abnormal Presentation:**				
	• Forceps delivery				
	• Vacuum delivery				
	• Breech delivery				
	• Multifetal delivery				
	• Cesarean section				
	• Assist with destructive operations				
7.	**Immediate Postnatal Care/Newborn Care:**				
	• Preparation of resuscitation unit				

Sl. No.	Subjects	Demonstration		Clinical	
		Date	Signature	Date	Signature
	• Resuscitation of newborn				
	• APGAR scoring				
	• Rooming in				
	• Immunization				
	• Initiation of immediate breastfeeding				
	• Maintain records and reports				
8.	**Providing Nursing Care to Postnatal Mother:**				
	• Preparing postnatal unit				
	• Postnatal assessment and examination of mother				
	• Immediate examination of newborn				
	• Perineal care				
	• Assist in breastfeeding				
	• Postnatal Examination—**BUBBLE-HE**				
	B-Breast examination assessment of breast and nipple illness				
	U-Uterus and abdominal examination				
	a. Measuring of abdominal girth, fundal height—assess the gestational age				
	b. Fundal palpation lateral and pelvic palpation				
	B-Bladder elimination—assess the urinary problems				
	B-Bowel elimination—assess for bowel elimination problems				
	L-Lochia				
	E-Episiotomy and perineal wound-check for wound healing				
	H-Homan's sign assessment				
	E-Check for the emotional status of the mother for any mood swings, anxiety and depression				
9.	**Newborn Examination:**				
	• Newborn assessment				
	• Cord and eye care				
	• Baby bath				
	• Immunization to baby				
	• Lactation management				
	• Registration of birth				
	• Maintenance of records and reports				
10.	**Nursing Care Newborn at Risk/NICU:**				
	• Newborn assessment				
	• Feeding of at risk neonates:				
	a. Katori spoon				
	b. Paladia				

Sl. No.	Subjects	Demonstration		Clinical	
		Date	Signature	Date	Signature
	c. Tube feeding				
	d. Total parenteral nutrition (TPN)				
	• Thermal management of neonates:				
	a. Kangaroo mother care				
	b. Incubator care				
	• Monitoring and care of neonates				
	• Administering medications				
	• Intravenous therapy				
	• Assisting with diagnostic procedures:				
	a. Ventilator care				
	b. Phototherapy				
	• Infection control protocols in the nursery				
	• Teaching and counseling of parents				
	• Maintenance of records				
11.	**Family Welfare Services:**				
	• Counseling techniques				
	• Insertion of IUD				
	• Motivation of planned parenthood				
	• Assist with tubectomy and vasectomy				
	• Teaching on use of family planning methods				
	• Arrange for and assist with family planning operations				
	• Maintenance of records and reports				
12.	**Nursing Care of Women with Gynecological Problems:**				
	• Assist with gynecological examination				
	• Assist and perform diagnostic and therapeutic procedures:				
	a. Colposcopy				
	b. Endocervical biopsy				
	c. Pap smear				
	d. Cystoscopy				
	• Teach women on breast-self examination (BSE)				
	• Health education on perineal hygiene and prevention of sexually transmitted infections				
	• Pre and postoperative care of women undergoing gynecological surgeries				
	• Menopause counseling				
13.	**Operative Obstetric Procedures:**				
	• Arrange and assist in MTP procedures				
	• Assist in ectopic delivery (laproscopy)				

Sl. No.	Subjects	Demonstration		Clinical	
		Date	Signature	Date	Signature
	• Arrange and assist in other surgical procedures				
	• Cesarean section: Care of mother and baby				

Requirements

Sl. No.	Completion of the requirements	Date	Signature
1.	Conducts ANC examination = 20		
2.	Perform vaginal examination = 05		
3.	Conducts normal delivery = 20		
4.	Episiotomy suturing = 05		
5.	Resuscitates newborn = 05		
6.	Provides PNC care = 20		
7.	Witness abnormal delivery = 05		
8.	Assist cesarean section = 02		
9.	IUCD insertion = 05		
10.	Family planning counseling = 02		
11.	Menopause counseling = 02		
12.	Assist in MTP = 05		
13.	Maintain drug book		
14.	Maintain the OT—obstetric instrument book		
15.	Documentation and completion of casebook recording		

Nursing Care Plan—Gynecology Ward

Sl. No.	Care Plan	Date	Signature
1.			
2.			

Case Study and Presentation/Ward Teaching

Sl. No.	Area	Date	Signature
1.	ANC		
2.	PNC		
3.	NICU		

Health Education

Date	Topic	AV aids	Place	Individual / group	Signature
			ANC ward		
			PNC ward		

Signature of Class Coordinator

Signature of the Principal

Drug Book

Sl. No.	Clinical area	Date of submission	Signature of supervisor
1.	ANC ward		
2.	Labor room		
3.	Operation theater		
4.	Postnatal ward		
5.	NICU		
6.	Family planning		
7.	Gynecology ward		

Signature of Class Coordinator **Signature of the Principal**

COMMUNITY HEALTH NURSING – II

Theory: 100 hours
Clinical: 168 hours

Sl. No.	*Subjects*	*Demonstration*		*Clinical*	
		Date	*Signature*	*Date*	*Signature*
1.	**Community Health Survey**				
2.	**Preparing Map of Community Area**				
3.	**Community Health Nursing Process**				
	• Assessment				
	• Community diagnosis				
	• Planning				
	• Implementation				
	• Evaluation				
4.	**Family Health Assessment**				
	• Maintenance of family folder				
5.	**Family Care: Home Adaptation of Common Procedures**				
	• Vital signs				
	• Dressing				
	• Baby bath				
	• Urine test: Sugar and albumin				
	Demonstration of Care				
	• Care of fever patient				
	• Oral rehydration therapy				
	Nutritional assessment				
	Home visit				
	Bag technique				
	Immunization/vaccination				
	Organize and Conduct Clinics				
	• Antenatal				
	• Postnatal				
	• Well baby clinic				
	• MCH clinic				
	• Family planning clinic				
	• Under five clinic				
	• School health clinic				
	• Health camps				
	• Geriatric clinic				
	• Immunization clinic				
	• Industrial clinic				
	• Handicapped home clinic				
	• Assisting in safe motherhood and safe childhood activities				

Sl. No.	*Subjects*	*Demonstration*		*Clinical*	
		Date	*Signature*	*Date*	*Signature*
	Screen, Manage and Referrals for:				
	• High risk mother ANC and PNC				
	• High risk neonates				
	• Accidents				
	• Emergencies				
	• Physical and mental illness				
	• Disabilities				
	Domiciliary Midwifery:				
	• Conducting antenatal examination at the clinic and ward				
	• Calculation of EDD/LMP				
	• Abdominal examination				
	• Inspection head-to-toe examination of the mother				
	• Examination of breast and nipple				
	• Examination of the abdomen:				
	a. Inspection				
	b. Measure the abdominal girth and fundal height				
	c. Estimate the gestational age				
	d. Palpation—fundal, lateral and pelvic examination				
	Assessment of risk status				
	• Immunization				
	• Teaching antenatal mothers				
	• Maintenance of antenatal records				
	• Check the vital signs				
	• Height				
	• Weight				
	• Provide antenatal advice				
	• Prepare family for safe delivery				
	• Administration of soap and water enema				
	• Maintain partograph				
	• Monitor fetal heart sounds				
	• Conducts home delivery				
	• Immediate care of newborn				
	• Meet the nutritional needs of mother and baby				
	• Resuscitate the newborn				
6.	**Postnatal Care in the Community:**				
	• Postnatal assessment and examination of mother				
	• Immediate examination of newborn				
	• Perineal care				
	• Assist in breastfeeding				
	• Postnatal Examination—**BUBBLE-HE**				

Sl. No.	Subjects	Demonstration		Clinical	
		Date	Signature	Date	Signature
	B-Breast examination assessment of breast and nipple illness				
	U-Uterus and abdominal examination				
	a. Measuring of abdominal girth, fundal height—assess the gestational age				
	b. Fundal palpation lateral and pelvic palpation				
	B-Bladder elimination—assess the urinary problems				
	B-Bowel elimination—assess for bowel elimination problems				
	L-Lochia				
	E-Episiotomy and perineal wound—check for wound healing				
	H-Homan's sign assessment				
	E-Check for the emotional status of the mother for any mood swings, anxiety and depression				
	• Warming				
	• Rooming in				
	• Assist in breastfeeding				
	• Cord care				
	• Immunization				
	• Postnatal care				
	a. Postnatal exercises				
	b. Postnatal advice				
	• Registration of birth and maintenance of birth records				
7.	**Family Planning and Family Welfare Services:**				
	• Oral contraceptives				
	• Injectable contraceptives				
	• Advise use of condoms—male and female				
	• Assisting in Cu-T insertion				
	• Assisting in permanent methods of sterilization				
	a. Tubectomy				
	b. Vasectomy				
	• Assisting in MTP/Abortion				
8.	**Vital Statistics:**				
	• Assisting and collecting vital statistics				
	a. Birth and death registers				
	b. Censes				
	• Participate in population survey				
	• Assist health professional in all health professional				
9.	**School Health Services:**				
	• School health assessment				
	• Identification of high-risk individuals				
	• Manage minor illnesses				

Sl. No.	*Subjects*	*Demonstration*		*Clinical*	
		Date	*Signature*	*Date*	*Signature*
	• Referrals for major illness				
	• Training and supervision of health workers				
10.	**Health Education:**				
	• Individual				
	• Family				
	• Group				
	• Community/mass				
11.	**Assist and Maintain Various Records and Reports:**				
	• ANC register				
	• Eligible couple register				
	• Immunization register				
	• Family planning register				
	• Stock register				
	• Family folder				
	• Birth and death register				
	• Writing community reports				
	• Epidemic reports				
	• Reports on National Health Program				
	• Maintain individual and family records				
	• Maintain administrative records				
12.	**Observational Visits:**				
	• School				
	• Industry				
	• Community mental health center				
	• National Family Planning Association of India				
	• National Institute of Tuberculosis				
	• Red Cross/WHO/UNICEF				
	• Professional bodies: TNAI/INC/State Nursing Council				
	• Isolation hospital				
	• Leprosarium				
	• Geriatric homes				
	• Remand homes				
	• Rehabilitation homes				
	• Homes for disabled				
	• Participates school health program and prepare a report				
	• Maintenance of daily diary in urban area				
	• Maintenance of daily diary in rural area				

Family Care Study and Family Profile

Sl. No.	*Area*	*Date of submission*	*Signature of supervisor*
	Urban		
	Rural		

Family Nursing Care Plan

Sl. No.	*Area*	*Date of submission*	*Signature of supervisor*
	Urban		
	Rural		

Standing Orders—Drug Book Maintained

Sl. No.	*Area*	*Date of submission*	*Signature of supervisor*
	PHC		
	Subcenter		
	Community health center		

Community Group Project

Sl. No.	*Area*	*Date of submission*	*Signature of supervisor*
	Urban		
	Rural		

Health Education

Sl. No.	*Clinical area*	*Topic*	*AV aids used*	*Place of presentation*	*Focus group*	*Date of submission*	*Signature of supervisor*
	Urban						
	Rural						

Community Health Nursing—Internship

Sl. No.	*Clinical area (6 weeks)*	*Date of completion*	*Signature of supervisor*
	Urban		
	Rural		

Signature of Class Coordinator **Signature of the Principal**

PRACTICAL EXAMINATION

MIDWIFERY AND GYNECOLOGICAL NURSING

Signature of Internal Examiner | Signature of External Examiner

Date: | Date:

Supplementary

Signature of Internal Examiner | Signature of External Examiner

Date: | Date:

COMMUNITY HEALTH NURSING – II

Signature of Internal Examiner | Signature of External Examiner

Date: | Date:

Supplementary

Signature of Internal Examiner | Signature of External Examiner

Date: | Date:

INTERNSHIP

Theory Subjects

Sl. No.	*Subjects*	*Hours*
1.	Nursing education	20
2.	Introduction to research and statistics	30
3.	Professional trends and adjustments	30
4.	Nursing administration and ward management	40
	Total	**120**

Clinical Areas

Sl. No.	*Clinical*	*Hours*
1.	Medical Surgical Nursing	258 (6 weeks)
2.	Community Health Nursing	258 (6 weeks)
3.	Child Health Nursing	86 (2 weeks)
4.	Midwifery and Gynecological Nursing	344 (8 weeks)
5.	Mental Health Nursing	86 (2 weeks)
	Total	1032 (24 weeks)

The students posted in the clinical areas should be accompanied by teaching faculty of the school

Night duty should be given in clinical area(s) in rotation.

* 43 hours per week for clinical and 5 hours per week for theory.

The same practice must be followed when student are posted for requisite clinical experience to affiliated hospital/agency/ institution

The nursing service personnel must actively participate in supervising, guiding and evaluating students in the hospital wards, health centers and in the community.

1:10 teacher student ratio to be maintained during the supervised clinical practice.

THIRD YEAR: PART-II (SCHOOL EXAMINATION)

Paper	*Subjects*	*Total Marks*	*Internal Marks*	*External Marks*	*Duration Exam*
1.	Nursing education and introduction to research and statistics	100	25	75	3
2.	Professional trends and adjustment, nursing administration and ward management	100	25	75	3

NURSING EDUCATION

Sl. No.	*Procedure*	*Date of presentation*	*Supervisors signature*
1.	**Utilizes Principles and Practice of Teaching**		
2.	**Teaching Methods:**		
	• Lecture method		
	• Demonstration method		
	• Discussion method		
	• Project method		
	• Laboratory method		
	• Problem solving method		
	• Nursing rounds		
	• Bedside clinic		
	• Nursing conferences		
3.	**Preparation of Lesson Plan**		
4.	**Preparation of Unit Plan/Course Plan**		
5.	**Understand the Responsibilities of Registered Nurse**		
6.	**Prepares and Utilizes the AV Aids in Health Teaching Classes:**		
	a. Audio aids		
	b. Visual aids		
	c. Projected aids		
	d. Non-projected aids		

Signature of Class Coordinator **Signature of the Principal**

INTRODUCTION TO RESEARCH AND STATISTICS

Sl. No.	*Research activities*	*Date*	*Supervisor signature*
1.	**Utilizes Steps in Research Process while Conducting Project Work and Report Writing**		
	• Introduction		
	• Background of the study		
	• Need for the study		
	• Statement of the problem		
	• Objectives of the study		
	• Operational definitions		
	• Variables		
	• Assumptions		
	• Limitations		
	• Hypothesis		
	• Conceptual framework		
	• Organization of report		
2.	**Review of Literature**		
	• Methodology		
	• Research approach		
	• Research design		
	• Setting of the study		
	• Statement of objectives		
	• Setting of the study		
	• Population		
	• Sampling technique and size		
	• Inclusive and exclusive criteria		
	• Content validity		
	• Development and description of tool		
	• Reliability		
	• Pilot study		
	• Data collection		
	• Plan for data analysis		
	• Discussion of findings		
	• Summary and conclusion		
	• Implications and recommendations		
	• Bibliography and annexures		
3.	**Assists in Clinical Research Activities**		
	• Uses different data collection techniques in gathering information		
	• Applies statistical methods in description of findings		
	• Descriptive statistics		
	• Inferential statistics		
	• Utilization of evidence-based practice in project work		
4.	**Research Report Presentation**		
5.	**Utilization and Communication of Research Findings**		

Signature of Internship In-charge

Date:

Signature of the Principal

Date:

NURSING ADMINISTRATION AND WARD MANAGEMENT

Sl. No.	*Clinical activity*	*Date*	*Signature of supervisor*
1.	**Principles of Clinical Administration**		
	• Supervision of cleanliness of the unit		
	• Delegation assignments of duties—staffs and students		
	• Preparation of duty roster		
	• Drug inventory:		
	a. General drugs		
	b. Narcotic drugs		
	• Ordering drugs, supplies and equipment		
	• Requisition for repair and replacement		
	• Equipment inventory		
2.	**Preparation of Job Description**		
	• Hospital staff:		
	a. Nursing superintendent		
	b. Departmental sister		
	c. Head nurse		
	d. Staff nurse		
	e. Nurse aides		
	• Educational Institutions:		
	a. Principal		
	b. Vice-Principal		
	c. Senior nursing tutor		
	d. Junior nursing tutor		
	e. Clinical instructor		
3.	**Maintenance of Leadership Styles**		
4.	**Organizing:**		
	• Orientation of new staff/student		
	• Clinical presentation/teaching		
	• Staff development programs		
	• Staff Welfare programs		
5.	**Maintenance of Record, Reports and Registers**		
	• Registers:		
	a. Census		
	b. Administration register		
	c. Discharge register		
	d. Drug register		
	• Reports:		
	a. Oral report		
	b. Written report		

Sl. No.	Clinical activity	Date	Signature of supervisor
	• Records:		
	a. Nurses records		
	b. Doctors records		
	• Observation of records maintained in the school		
6.	**Preparation of Evaluation Tools**		
	• Patient care evaluation		
	• Student evaluation		
	• Staff evaluation		
7.	**Organizing Educational Tours to Various Institutions**		

Signature of Internship In-charge

Date:

Signature of the Principal

Date:

Requirements

Sl. No.	Requirements	Topic	Date	Signature
1.	Medical Surgical Nursing-5 Care Notes/Care Study			
2.	Community Health Nursing-3 Family Care Studies			
3.	Psychiatric Nursing-3 Care Notes/Care Study			
4.	Pediatric Nursing-3 Care Notes/Care Study			
5.	Midwifery and Gynecological Nursing-5 Care Notes			

Signature of the Class Coordinator

Date:

Signature of the Principal

Date:

Supplementary

1. Signature of Internal Examiner

   Date:

2. Signature of Internal Examiner

   Date:

1. Signature of External Examiner

   Date:

2. Signature of External Examiner

   Date:

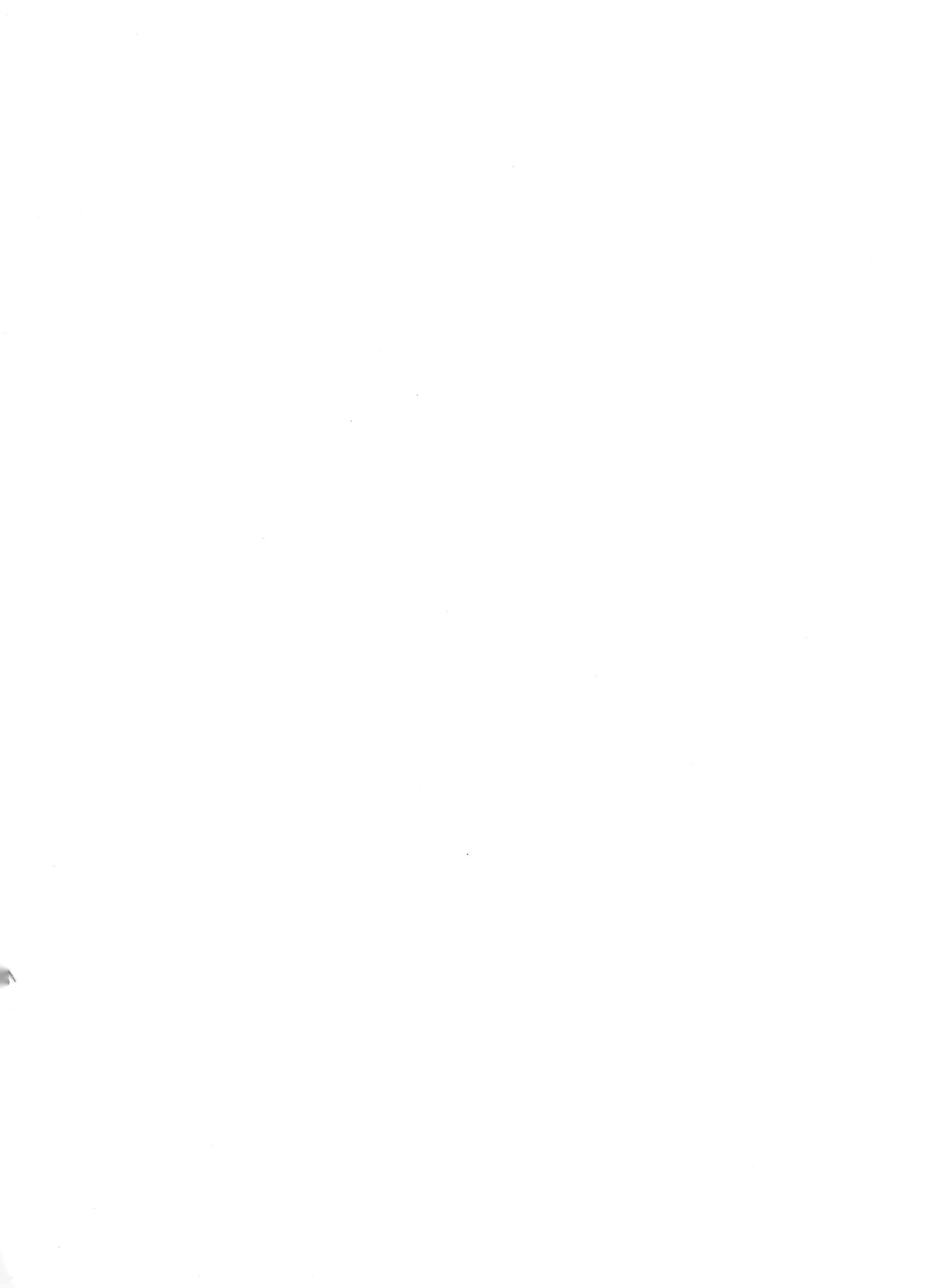